THIS PANDEMIC

WE MUST

END IT!

By Rose Marie B. Wolford-Zabala

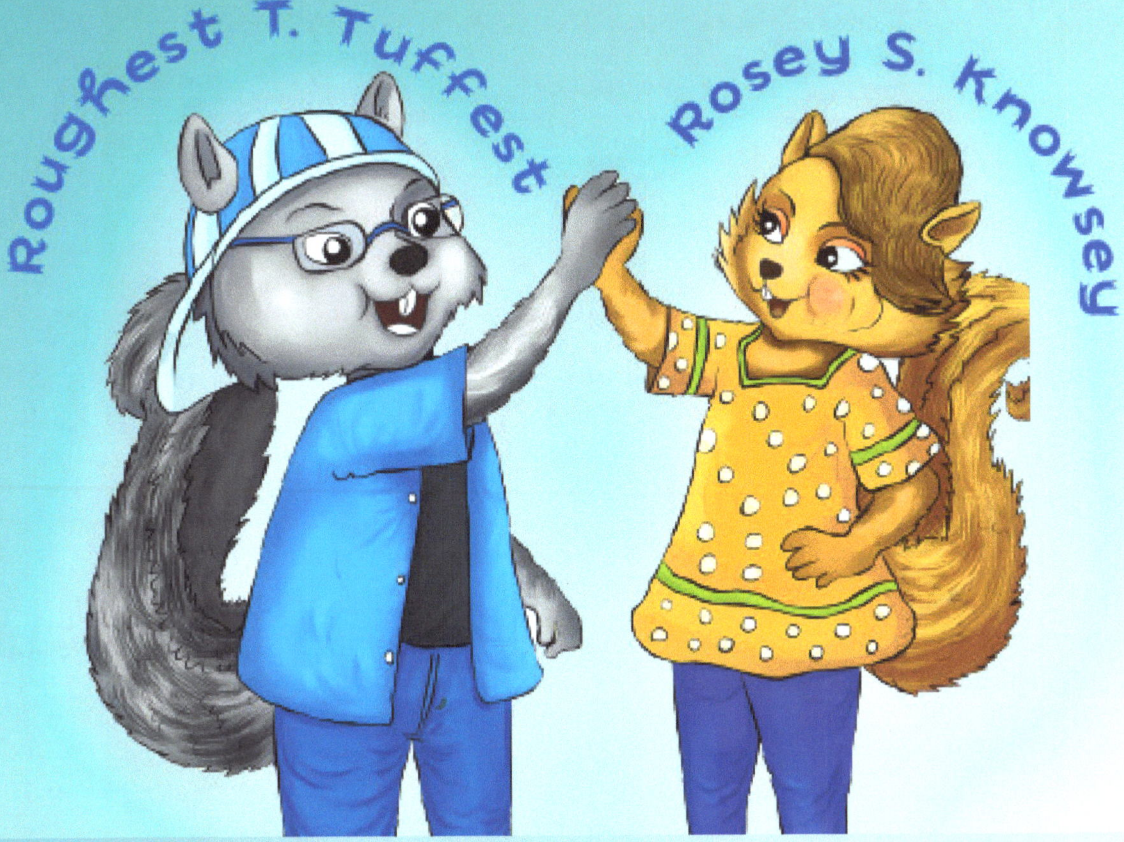

Rose Marie B. Wolford-Zabala

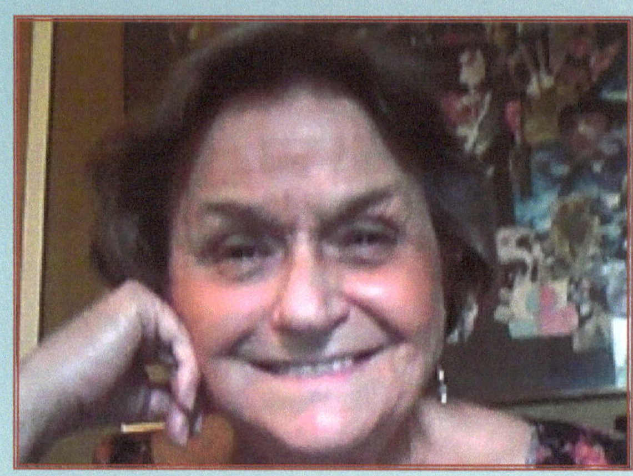

To the reader and "read to" of this book:
Currently throughout our world
A presence of divisions hurled
That tries to rip the heart and mind
Destroy the spirit of mankind
'through division, indecision'
but we must rise to fight
our differences 'stressed' in this plight
By focusing on ALL we share
with 'binding strength and right' UNITE!

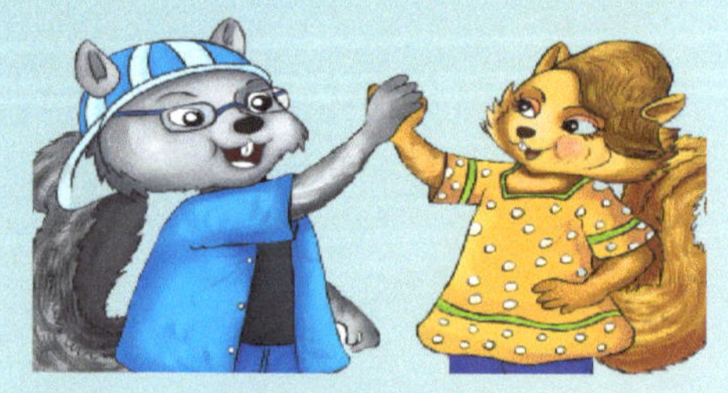

Special thanks to
Dolores (DD), French & Vilma Wolford

ISBN: **9798598835562**

Carrie Campbell, Counselor/SUDCCII #6873, Palmdale, Ca. U.S.A.
Dr. Billy C. Lawrence, Theologian & Author, Colorado Springs, CO. U.S.A.
Susan Markebjer - Säfström, Behavioral/Counselor: Youth & Early Intervention,
Stockholm Vallentuna, Sweden

I'm grateful
to my parents
John and Katherine
Zabala who taught me
integrity. Many thanks to
my supportive endorsers who
believed in me and the subject
matters addressed in this book series.
Special thanks to my son Robb Wolford who
often encouraged and went through "huge"
amounts of collaborative and most likely often
frustrating editing. Thanks to all my sons and their
children . As well as, all the children who have always
inspired my spirit to keep on no matter what! And, of course
Father God, Who was and is and always will be I AM, that I AM

and
YHWH
for His
gifts
for
all

Grateful thanks~Colleen Hanks!
Special thanks to Shada Baduwi
who brought the characters alive in
the cooperative/collaborative efforts
illustrating and designing of this book:
ABC Education Materials and Training

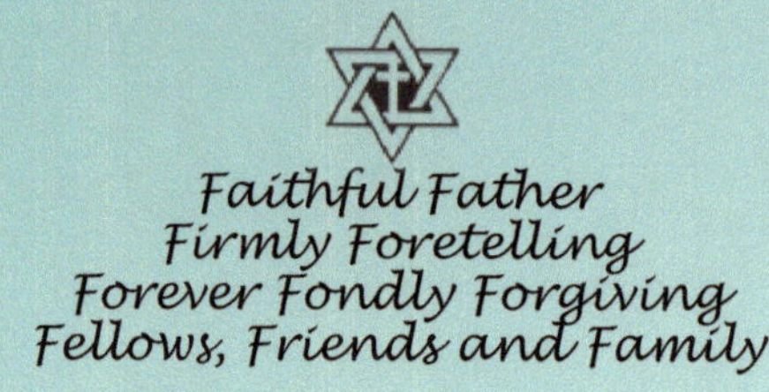

Rose Marie Wolford-Zabala is a Cognitive Behaviorist, Special Educator/Advocate and former Children Social Worker. Her experiences moved her to write the rhyming book series addressing current social-emotional, familial and environmental issues today experienced by families. At this point in time the first of 16 books to be published.

Rosey so Nosey and Roughest the Toughest series addressing:

Domestic Violence	Reading	Bullying
Divorce/Separation	Teamwork	Pollution
Family diversity	Hazards of Lying	Substance Abuse
Fear/Anxiety/Secrets	Stealing/Wrong conclusions	Water Conservation
Siblings fighting/reconciliation	Friends fighting and forgiving	Health Crisis/Safety

Rosey loved to explore and learn of "new things"
Not afraid of things different, while others did cling
To the same, not arrange, often shying from change
Due to fear of UNKNOWN and things out of range.
Rosey searched for the new and embraced this new treasure
Shared "discovers" with others for it brought her much pleasure
Roughest, her best friend helps find a way
Yes, they CAN find solutions and help save the day!
Let's all read together find what happened before
For the problem in store and we'll learn all the more
How Rosey and Roughest push problems away
Let's find out! All about...see what happened that day.

Walking down the street…

Rosey went to meet

Her good friend Roughest…

They are hoping to defeat…

This ever growing spiral

of people in denial…

Though cases going viral

With this
virus
that defies us!

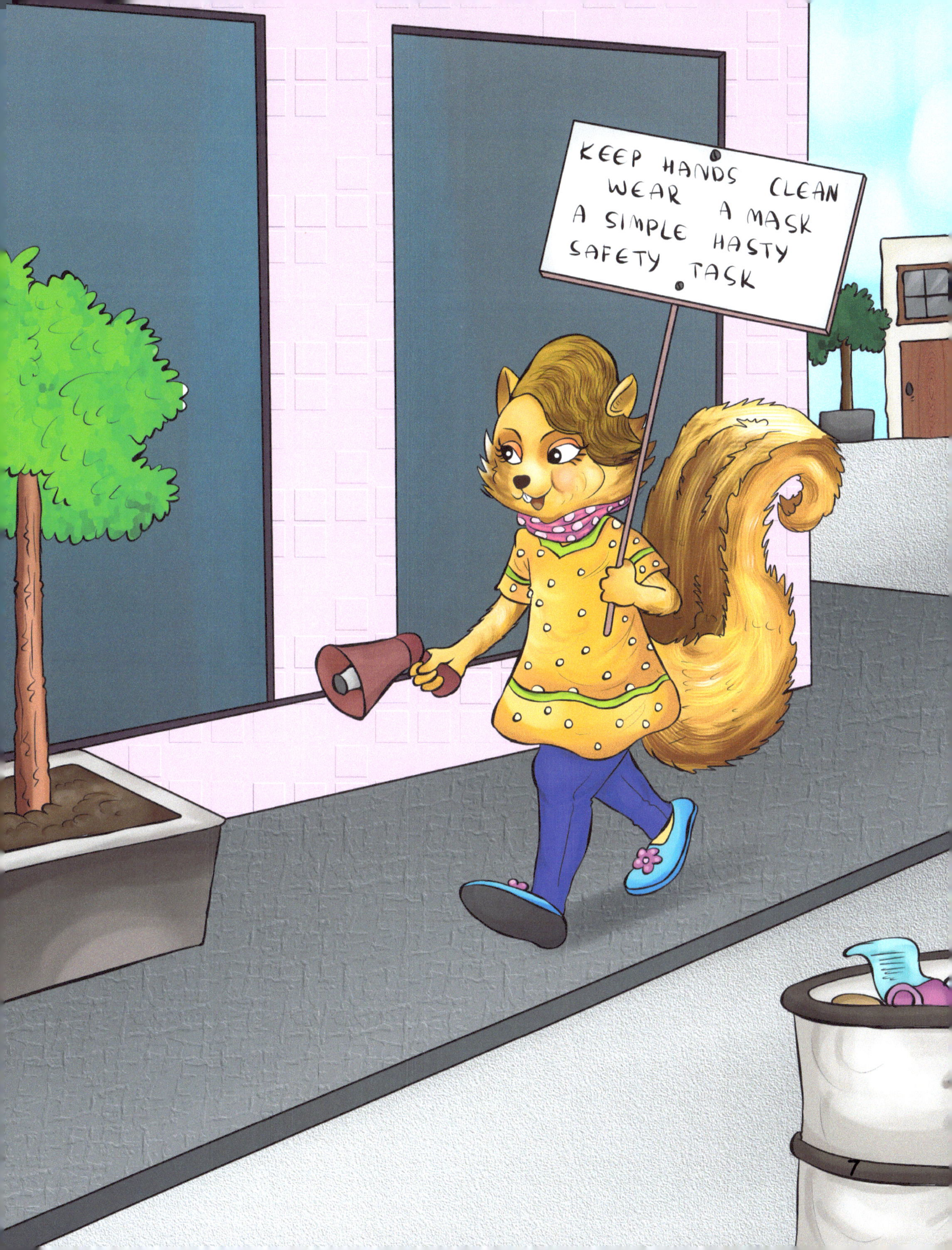

KEEP HANDS CLEAN
WEAR A MASK
A SIMPLE HASTY
SAFETY TASK

Rosey noticed a large group.…

Holding signs within their troop

What she saw dropped her jaw!

So MANY there to push resistance

To pleas and calls for social distance,

Banned united with consistence

*Not to keep **the**
'distance task'.*

Not to wear 'mandated
mask'.
Such insistence to
resistance!

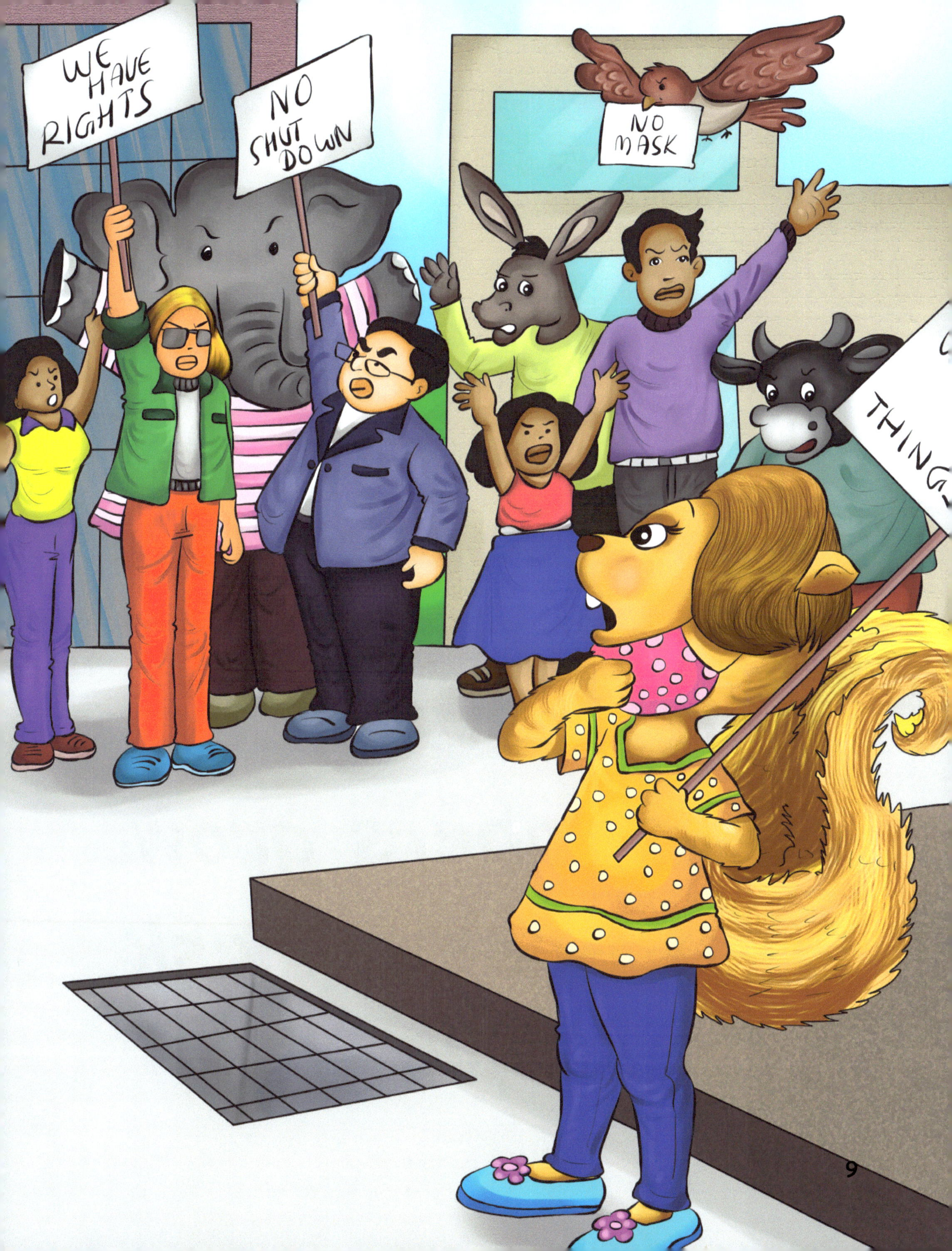

9

They gathered round not
wearing masks
Though signs were posted
'round with facts:
'Wear a mask in public places'
'Wash your hands and cover faces'

**This guards against and helps to ease,
the dread and spread of this disease!**

*The facts impact
as numbers grow.
Just wear a mask,
a simple task!*

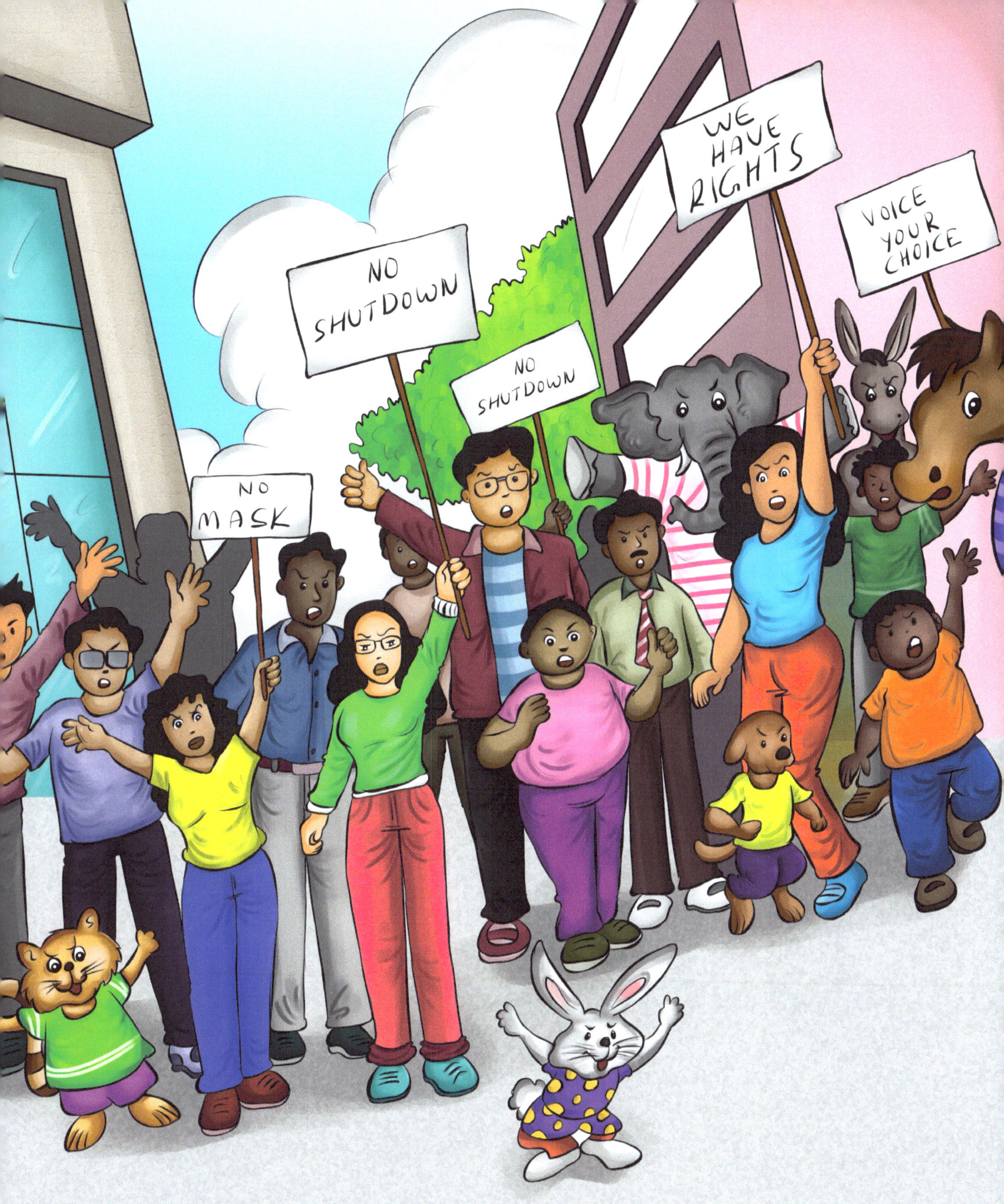

NO SHUTDOWN
NO SHUTDOWN
NO MASK
WE HAVE RIGHTS
VOICE YOUR CHOICE

A 'road to tow'
for all to show
Respect for all
both friend and foe

The *virus* moves
within the air....

and who **IT** harms

IT doesn't care!

RIGHT NOW
there is
NO CURE
FOR SURE!
BEWARE
INCAUTION!
USE
PRECAUTION!

It's not as **hard**
as some may think.
Who **DEFY - DENY** and
CAUSE A STINK!

Who **feel** that they
should have *their right*
to disagree... **not**
JOIN THE FIGHT!

Though **DOING SUCH**
is **CAUSING MUCH**
DISTRESS and STRESS...
It's **QUITE A MESS!**
For **DOING SO**
the **VIRUS GROWS**
It's **SUCH A CRIME!**
While ***NUMBERS CLIMB!***
A crime against humanity
for selfish rights...
INSANITY!

Roughest walking down the street

To join his friend and help defeat

To meet and come up with a plan

To help and end

this NO MASK BAN!

Of those who want to heap defeat...

the calls for "masks and distance keep"

To those **who offer no assistance**

To those who show a great

resistance!

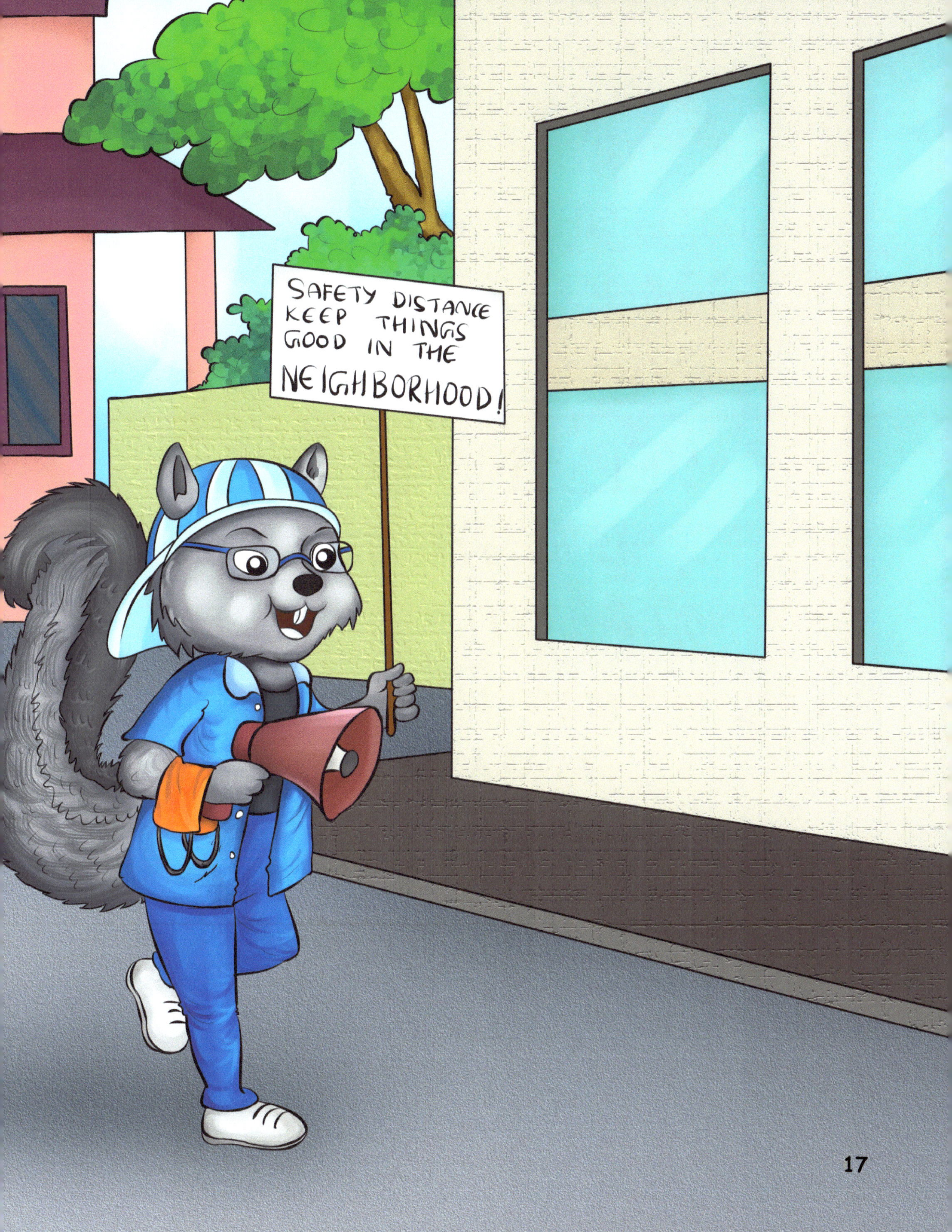

17

Insisting that they have **their right**...
NOT TO FOLLOW IN THIS FIGHT!
Rosey and Roughest saw the crowd...

YELLING OUT,
YELLING LOUD!

'We have the right...
NOT to LISTEN or ABIDE!
We have freedom! We have pride!
To **MASK UP**

HINDERS LIBERTY.

We all have rights both you and me'

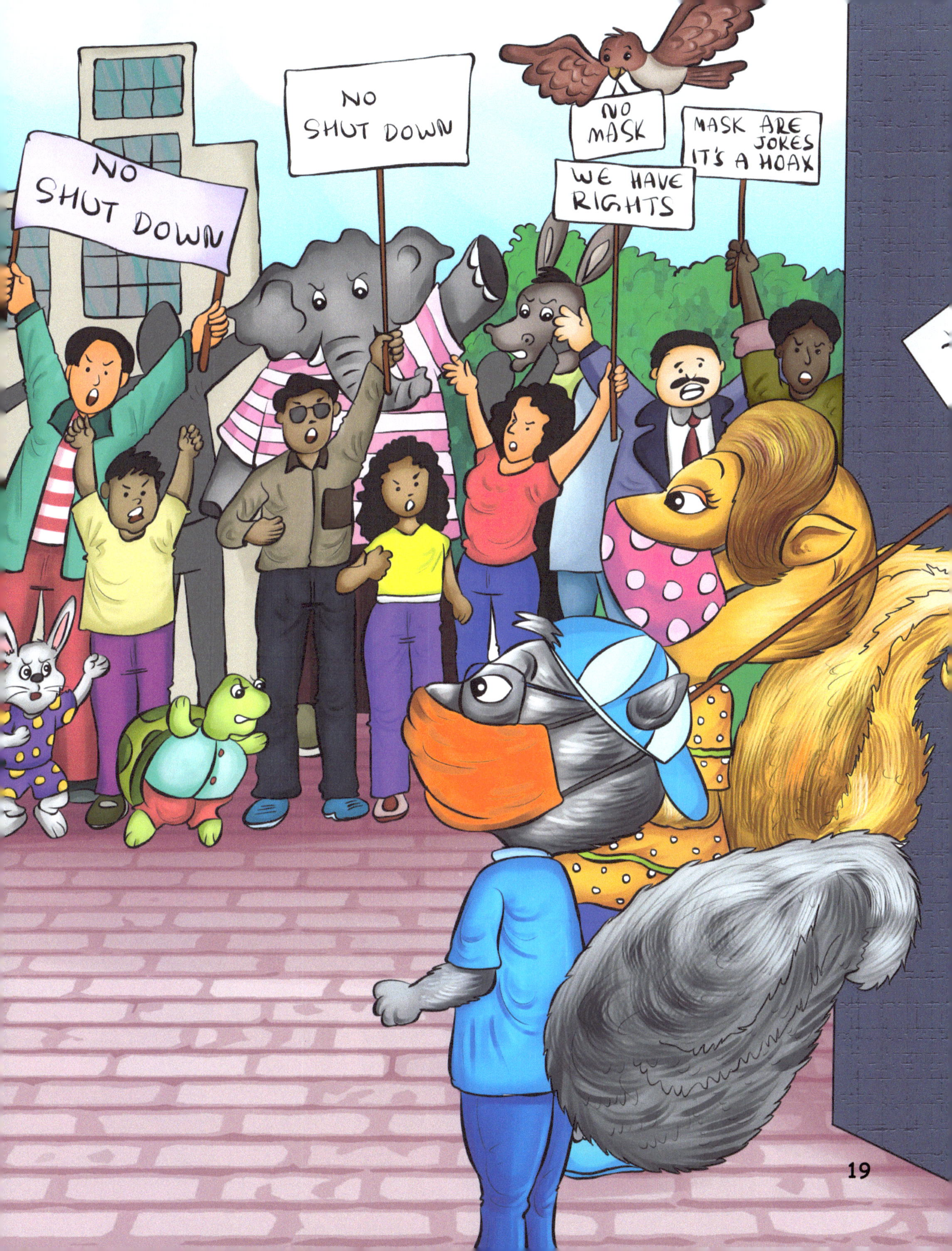

NO SHUT DOWN
NO SHUT DOWN
NO MASK
WE HAVE RIGHTS
MASK ARE JOKES IT'S A HOAX

Rosey and Roughest **masked** did ask,

a question to the crowd did cast:

'Does this *include* that you *intrude*

on *other's rights and their belief?*

The scientific facts achieved...

not wearing masks has caused

MUCH GRIEF!

Not wearing masks with others 'round,

harms, alarms and numbers bound!

What about the rights of all?

Is *rude, crude bullying*

a rightful call?'

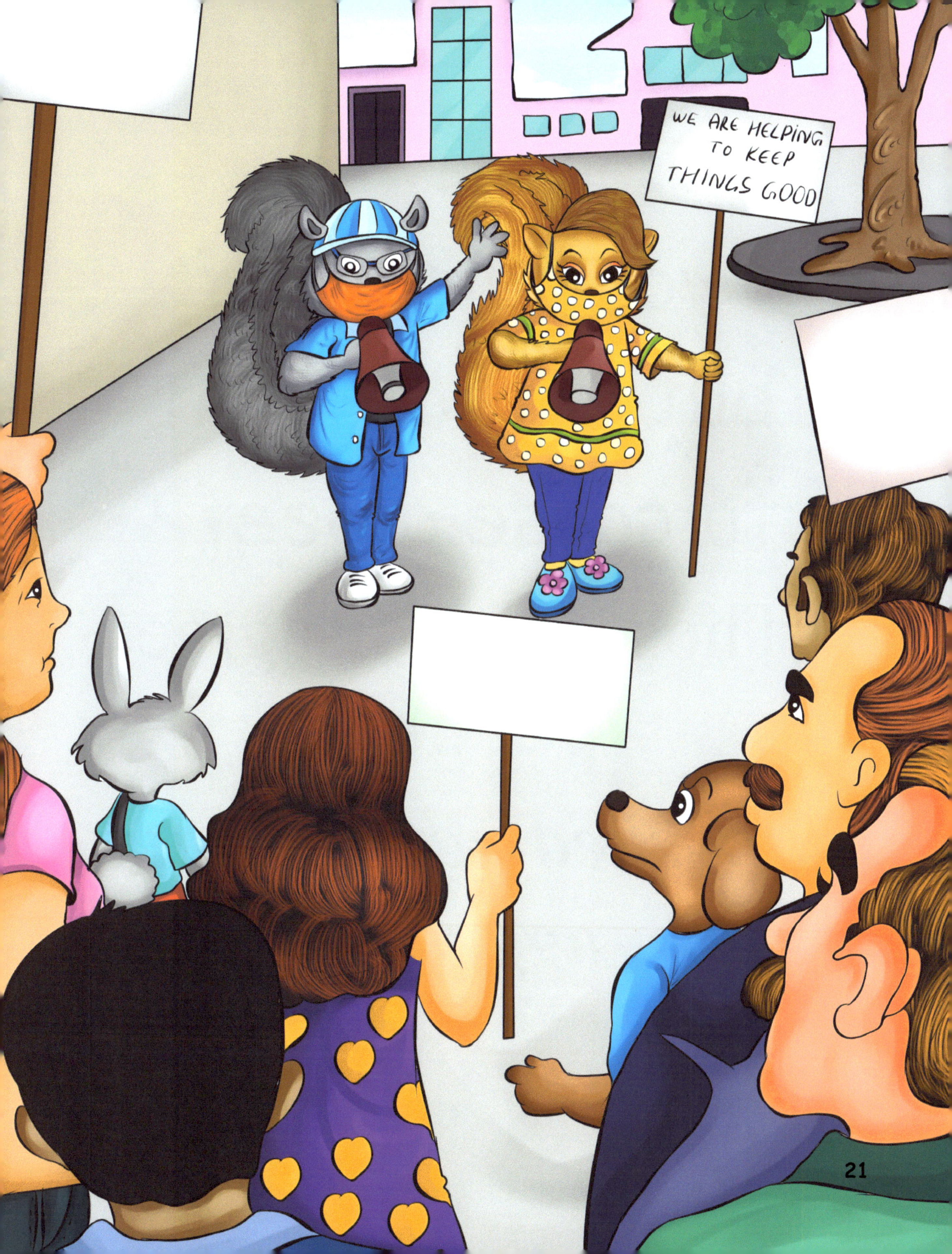

WE ARE HELPING
TO KEEP
THINGS GOOD

'You may have
your disbelief
but is that right
to cause a beef?
Those who disagree
perceive
*unmasked actions cause
aggrieve!*'

22

'Leads to people spreading sickness...

RAPID

RATES

with

SUDDEN

QUICKNESS'

'*Coughing* and *choking*
propelling in air

This **known virus-**
this **known fear**

Without a mask it freely flows,
Affecting others as it goes
Circulating with the wind
To find a host around the bend

A simple mask
helps do the task

To bring the cycle
to an end!'

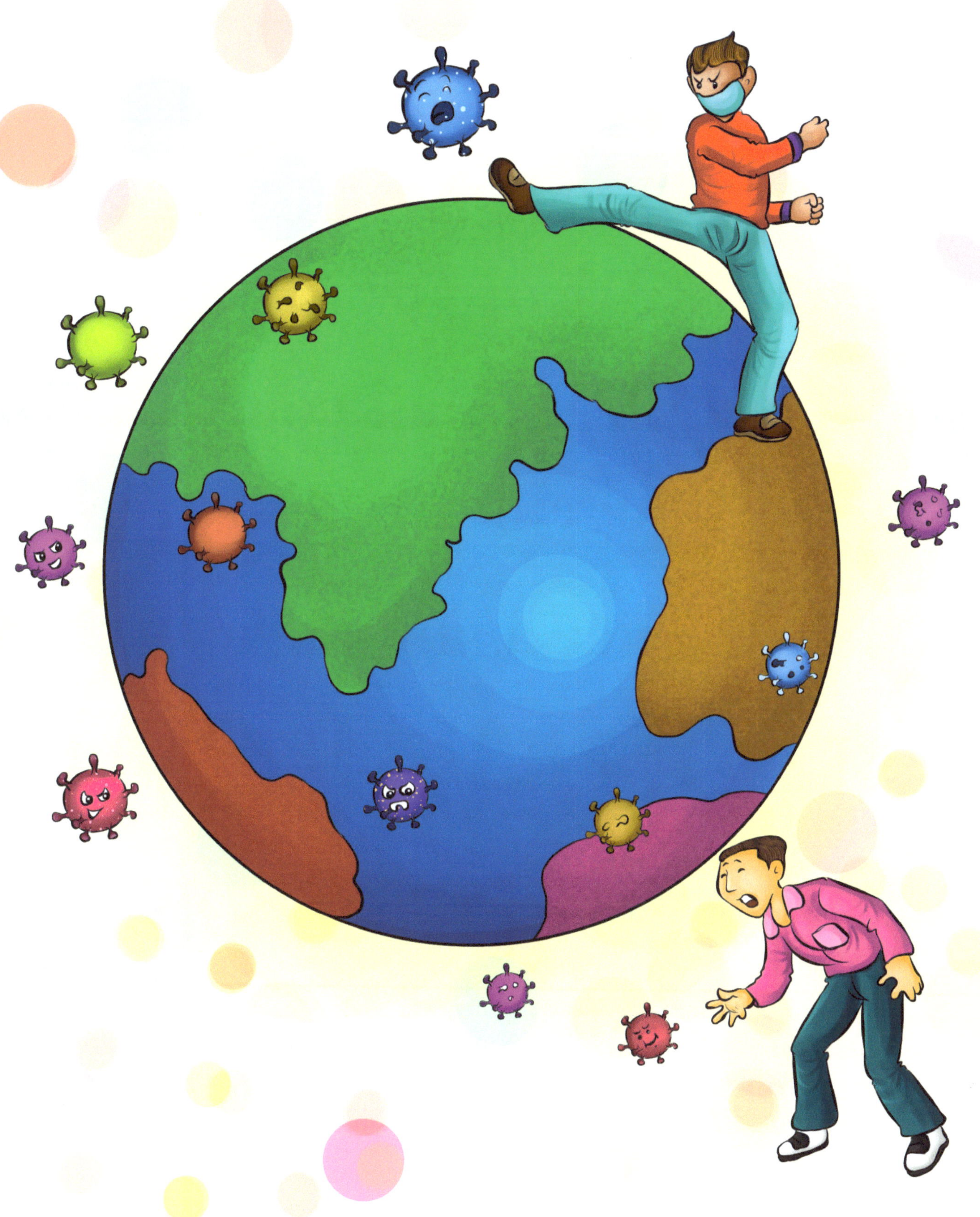

'The safety guides, they are a plea.

It hinders no one's liberty!

It is a plea for all you see to work together and be free

To once again have

NORMALCY

to BUILD up our

ECONOMY!'

'Not a **POLITICAL,
CYNICAL** scheme!
It's a way to end this viral stream!
It's **NOT A JOKE!**
It's **NOT A HOAX!**
It **GUIDES TO COAX**
and
SAVE ALL FOLKS!'

Rosey and Roughest
NEED

your HELP
To END...
THIS WHELP!
THIS HYPE!
THIS
YELP!

Rosey and Roughest gave

FINAL PLEAS...
to end
'THIS SEIGE'
Decrease!
Bring
Peace...

'YES, WE ALL
ARE DIFFERENT...
'UNIQUELY
CREATED'

YET, technology **GROWS** and **ZOOMS** ...NOT DATED!

NOW *at times...*'Face to Face' can't be...

but **NOW we CAN** 'meet' **VIRTUALLY!**

With loved ones, friends and family.'

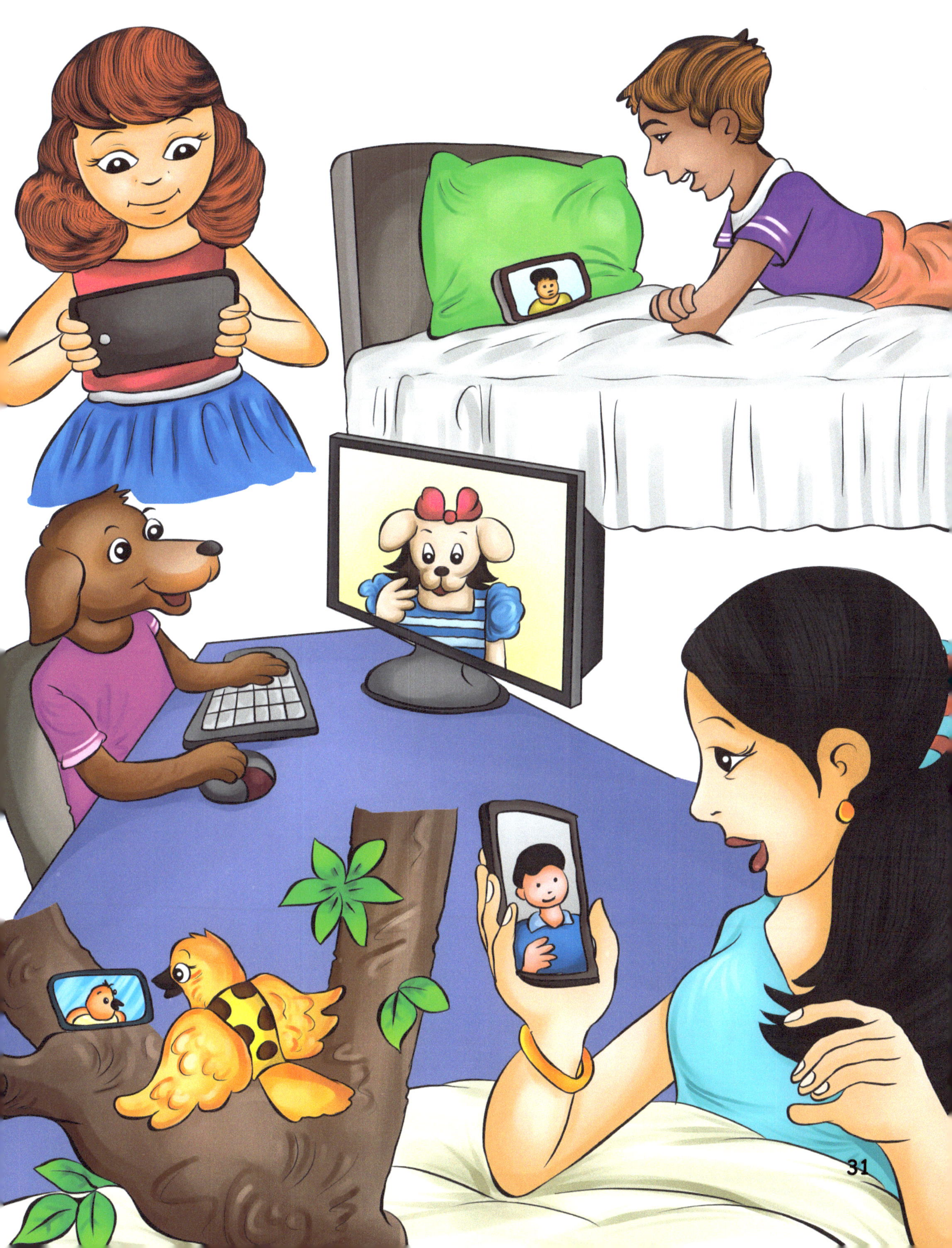

'Let's stop this

hyped up

raised

tsunami

threatening all

from A-Z

Threatening all

both you and me!'

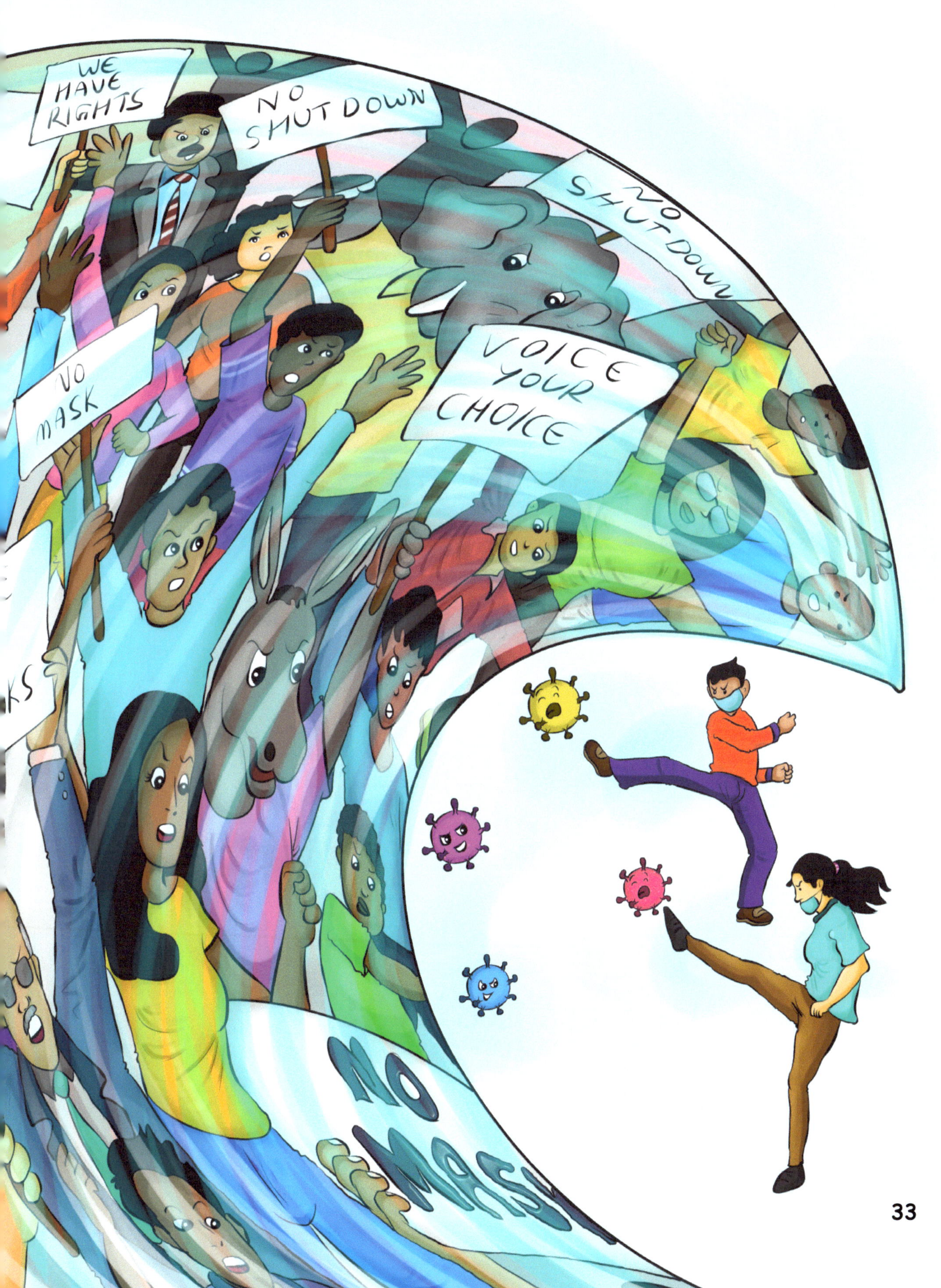

WE HAVE RIGHTS
NO SHUT DOWN
NO SHUT DOWN
NO MASK
VOICE YOUR CHOICE
KS
NO MASK

'For soon **vaccines will
come around...**
but **our defenses cannot ground!**
We must continue safety guards...
until our numbers can be sound!

To know **for sure** the
vaccine's working…

our **safety measures**

can't be shirking!

Respecting science and each other,

Disciplining one another

Soon we'll conquer it as one,

PULL TOGETHER

MAKE IT RUN!'

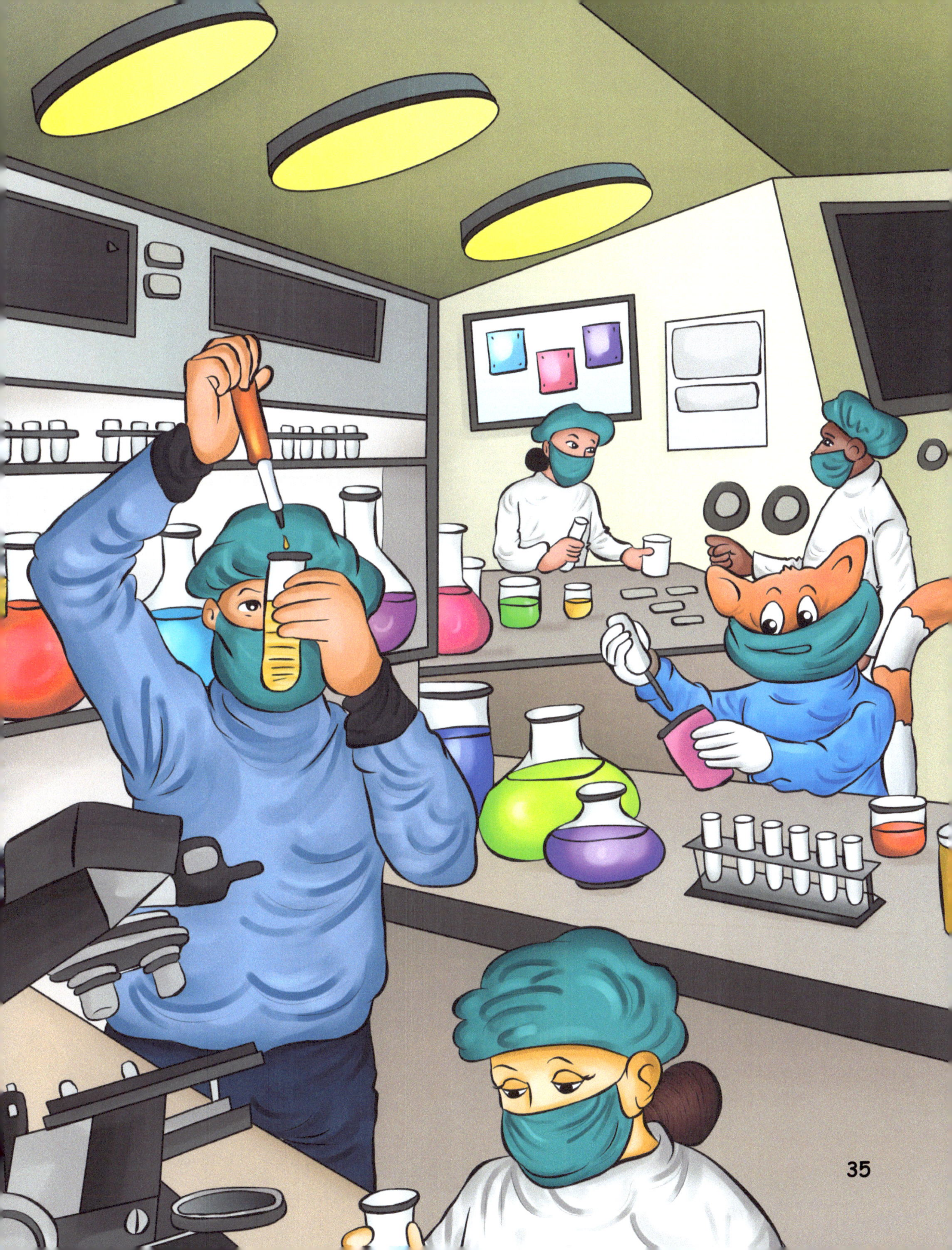

One day
history will show
WE KNEW
'what and how' to go.
We knew how to
'send the trend'
and WE KNEW
how to
'make it

mend'

We DID UNITE
'in right to fight'
THIS
HORRID
VIRUS
HAD TO END!

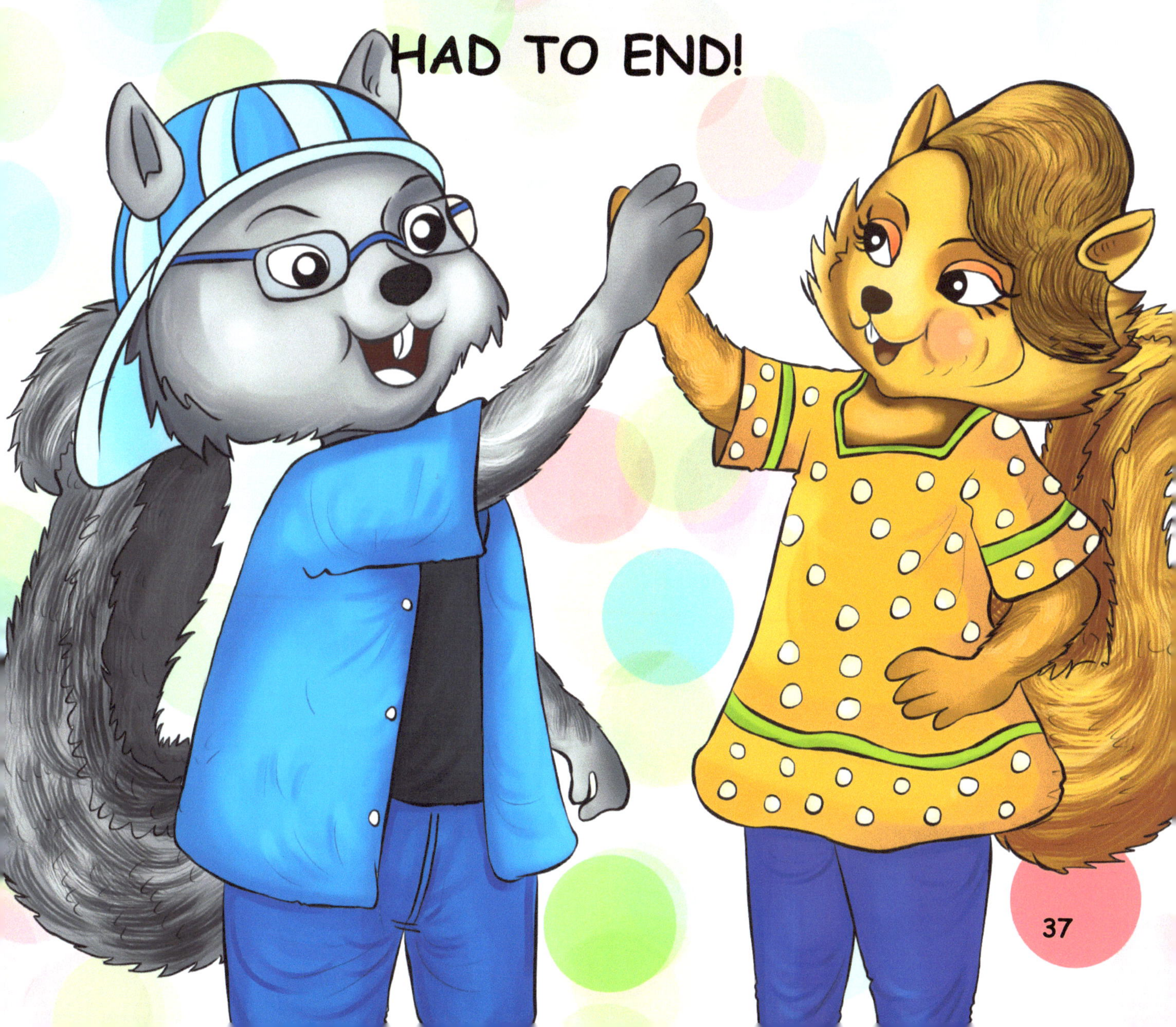